Praise for The Healing Power of Doodling

"Your 'Sacred Doodles' are profound renderings of the whimsy and the wit of the creative unconscious. Drawing, as they do on the kinesthetic sense, which itself is attached to the subtle muscular knowings of our liminal life, you have brought forth something that has huge appeal."

–Jean Houston, Ph.D., scholar, philosopher and researcher in Human Capacities

"*The Healing Power of Doodling* is a wonderfully fun book. When I was developing my effortless mindfulness practices while working as a psychotherapist in Brooklyn I would doodle in between clients. It gave me a way of expressing something that is beyond words, yet is embodied and wanting to be shared. I know you will enjoy Carol's gift to us all."

–Loch Kelly, author of *The Way of Effortless Mindfulness*

"As a stressed out mom of two and full-time 3rd grade teacher, Carol's program has been an island of calm in my otherwise hectic life. Doodling has allowed me and my students to destress, regroup, and refocus. Thank you Carol! You have changed our lives for the better."

–Linda Cornejo, School Teacher

"Brilliant...an important contribution to integrative medicine. A book that anyone with a serious interest in the field ought to read."

–Tom Gordon, Retired Executive Vice President of Cedars-Sinai Health System

"Carol Edmonston takes us by the hand and gently introduces us to the natural mindfulness of our inner artist. Through simple doodle prompts the author shows us how to destress, center and calm ourselves in a world full of challenges."

    –Lucia Capacchione, Ph.d, Art Therapist, author and pioneer in Expressive Art Therapy

"This highly original contribution can help you touch your inner resources leading to health and well being. I cannot imagine anyone who would not benefit."

    –Larry Dossey M.D., Former Executive Editor of the peer-reviewed journal of Alternative Therapies in Health and Medicine. *New York Times* bestselling author and advocate of the role of the mind in health and the role of spirituality in healthcare

"In our modern world, kids experience more anxiety and stress than ever before. With an assault on their attention span, Carol's doodling book provides a tremendous benefit to their well being guiding them to peace, mindfulness and an exploration of their imagination."

–Eva Jensen, M Ed, Studio Teacher, International Alliance of Theatrical Stage Employees (IATSE)

"Carol's message is both honest and inspirational. Simply put, she reminds us that life is precious and that we should try to honor and value it by the way we live our lives every day..."

    –Ambassador George M. Staples, Retired Diplomatic Advisor to The Supreme Allied Commander Europe NATO

"*The Healing Power of Doodling* gives you a simple way to relax and become centered in just a few minutes....and all you need is a pen!"

    –Steve Harrison, Co-founder of the National Publicity Summit

The Healing Power of Doodling

MINDFULNESS THERAPY TO DEAL WITH
STRESS, FEAR & LIFE CHALLENGES

The Healing Power of Doodling

CAROL EDMONSTON
THE DOODLE LADY™

Bindu Publications

Bindu Publications

700 E. Birch St., Suite 264

Brea, CA 92822

ISBN: 978-0-9700684-2-2

Library of Congress Control Number: 2020903006

Cover Design: Christy Collins, Constellation Book Services

Editor: David Aretha

Copy Editor: Christopher Edmonston

Printed in the United States of America

Art opens the closets, airs out the cellars and attics.
It brings healing...

–Julia Cameron, *The Artist's Way*

Introduction

Let's face it — stress isn't going away! If you are like most people, you may be experiencing more stress in your everyday life trying to juggle this and that — professionally and personally. But that doesn't mean you need to allow yourself to become paralyzed by stress, or let it build up and become chronic, which can compromise your immune system and, in turn, negatively impact your overall health and well-being.

What makes one person sail through a challenging or chaotic event, while another struggles, depends, in part, upon one's coping strategies. Whether our challenges are great or small, they can serve as a springboard for growth and transformation. We have a choice. We can choose to discover their gifts, or bury our heads in the ground and pretend everything will be fine.

I had my own frightening experience with fear and anxiety when I was first diagnosed with breast cancer in 1995, and then again exactly two years later in my other breast. My initial thoughts were filled with all those scary "what if" scenarios, wondering if I was going to die, if my son was going to lose his mother, my husband his wife. I wondered how something like this could be happen to me, as I ate well, exercised and meditated every day. I initially felt frozen and scared.

Then something magical happened one day while I nervously waited for a doctor's appointment. I had asked the nurse for pen and paper to pass the time and started to doodle. Before I knew it, I began to feel a sense of calm and peace. The more I doodled, the calmer I felt. And in no time, this seemingly frivolous and mindless activity had become a daily spiritual practice — an open-eyed meditation — one that helped me stay focused in the present moment and out of those scary unknown tomorrows.

Doodling is more than just a mindless and frivolous activity of distraction. It can help access the body's healing wisdom and allow your spirit to rest, recover and regroup.

I want to share this Sacred Doodles Method with you and hope it will serve as a vehicle to inner calm as you navigate through your busy and sometimes unpredictable lives. Plus, doodling is fun, no art skills are necessary, and you can do it most anywhere. All you need is pen and paper.

May your journey through this book inspire you to become the artist of your own life one doodle at a time. Let's have fun!

Carol

The Doodle Lady™

To help you get started, I've included a few of my original outlines and the finished doodles. At first glance the outlines look rather chaotic and messy, just as life can be at times with events that pop out of nowhere and catch us off guard. That's when we need to push the pause button and take a deep breath.

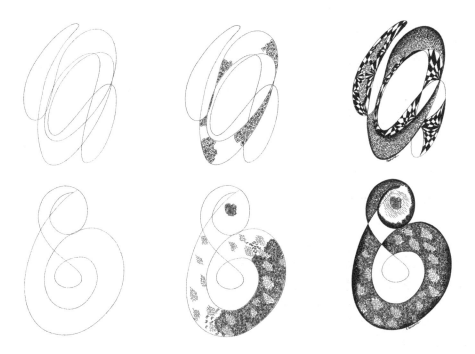

Using the Sacred Doodles Method you'll learn how to shift gears, quiet your mind and cultivate a sense of trust and faith, not only in a creative process, but in life, as well. You'll see how outer chaos can dissolve into something of beauty as you journey from beginnings, to middles, to endings and how they fit together. The key is letting go of your hook into results and outcomes. Remember — life is about the journey, not the destination, and it begins at the end of your comfort zone. Let's begin!

Sacred Doodles Method

Use a clean sheet of paper or the blank space on the next page to create your doodle outline. You can use colored or non-colored pens or pencils.

⌘ Take a good posture. Close your eyes and take a few deep breaths — a deep breath in and a long breath out, letting go of all the excess mind chatter going on, those thoughts outside this present moment, all those "what was" and "what's yet to come" events. If you have a lot of chatter going on, perhaps worried about a meeting that didn't go as planned, the kids, the in-laws or anything else, gently place those thoughts in an imaginary straw basket that's on the floor next to you labeled "My Stress Basket."

⌘ Now, bring your attention back to this moment as you open your eyes.

⌘ In the time it takes to count to three, and without lifting the pen off the paper, let your pen wander randomly in one continuous motion trying to begin and end your doodle outline at the same point. Don't try and create anything you can imagine in your mind (a house, tree or animal). Surrender to the freedom of not knowing what the result will look like. Trust the process — trust this creative middle. Whatever ends on the paper will be perfect! Give it a whirl.

⌘ How did that feel? Did you feel at ease trusting a spontaneous creative moment, or perhaps a bit uncomfortable surrendering to the unknown? Now try another doodle outline. Did you feel more at-ease? Take a moment and write down your experience under each doodle outline.

Doodle Outline #1:

Doodle Outline #2:

Now it's your turn to create a new doodle outline on the next page and fill it in with whatever comes to mind — dots, circles, lines, hearts. Spend the next 20-30 minutes and let your imagination be your guide. You may use plain or colored paper. There are no rules! Trust your intuition and don't worry about "what" you create — just have fun "creating."

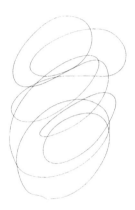 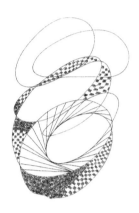 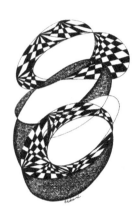

Do not overthink. Give yourself permission to trust your intuition and surrender to the process with little concern about the end result. You can use either black ink or colored pens/pencils. Art is all about being able to express yourself without judgement. If you like, you can add some quiet background music such as instrumental Native American flute or Celtic harp. However, it's preferably not to have the television on or other distractions that can easily pull you out of a quiet space. Let this activity become a healing ritual, as it nourishes your spirit from the inside out.

As you doodle, be mindful of any mental chatter that may be pulling you out of the present moment into other time zones. If that happens, gently bring yourself back to the present by taking a few deep breaths in and few long breaths out. Breathe in a sense of calm, and breathe out anxiety or worry. Focus on that space in between the in-breath and out-breath — that's the portal to the sacred where the noisy outer world melts into calm.

[doodle page]

Just as in life, things don't always make sense or present themselves in a tidy, neat package, but it doesn't mean you should judge, avoid or push them aside. In times like that it's important to take a reflective pause and a few deep breaths before you take the next step.

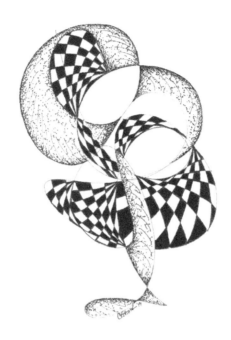

Remember, you may not have a choice as to what comes into your life, but you do have a choice in how you respond. On the next page, take a few moments and write down some of the challenges you may currently be experiencing and how you're dealing with them, or look at past events and choices you made. Did you take to time to quiet your mind and reflect on possible solutions before deciding what to do, or did you react with a knee-jerk response to the anxiety and stress? The important lesson is to learn something about yourself without judgment so you can choose differently tomorrow. Connect with the wellspring of wisdom you have within without continuing to dwell on "what was."

[journal page]

_____

_____

_____

_____

_____

_____

_____

_____

_____

Doodling is about wonderment.

It is more than just an activity of distraction.
It can take you to a deeper space within
where you can rest within the silence
      of your heart and
connect with the seeds of faith,
      courage and hope.

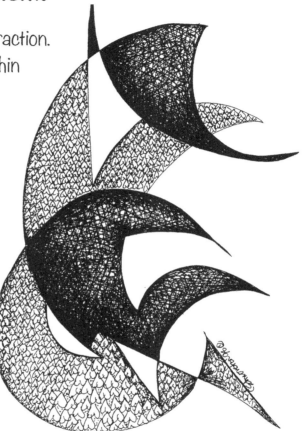

[doodle page]

Now that you've completed your doodle, take some time and write down how the process felt and what you learned about yourself. Were you able to surrender to the moment with ease — to trust and have faith in the creative process with little regard to end result? Did you feel a sense of relaxation — a sense of peace and calm within? If not, what did you experience? If your mind wandered to worldly concerns, were you able to bring yourself back to the present moment with relative ease?

_____

_____

_____

_____

Can you see any parallel between how you engage with a wandering mind while you doodle, and a wandering mind while you interact with the outside world? An undisciplined mind can easily take you down a path filled with stress and anxiety when you find yourself dwelling in the "if onlys" or the "what ifs".

It is by anchoring yourself in the present moment where you can connect with your higher self and the wellspring of wisdom and inner guidance you long for to help as you navigate through challenges of everyday life. This is the power of using doodling.

And...the good news is there are no mistakes when doodling! One day you may enjoy looking at it horizontally, while the next day you may like it vertically.

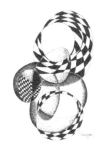

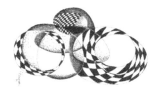

[doodle page]

Every doodle is unique just like a snowflake — a one-of-a-kind. You don't need to compare it to anyone else's, or have it professionally analyzed. Simply take refuge in knowing your doodle reflected a peaceful present moment where you took the time to nourish and nurture your spirit.

Use the following blank pages to create more doodles following the Sacred Doodles Method:

In the time it takes to count to three, let your pen wander randomly in one continuous motion trying to begin and end your outline at the same point without lifting the pen off the paper. Don't try and create anything you can imagine in your mind. Surrender to the freedom of not knowing what the result will look like. Trust the process — the creative middle. Whatever ends on the paper will be perfect!

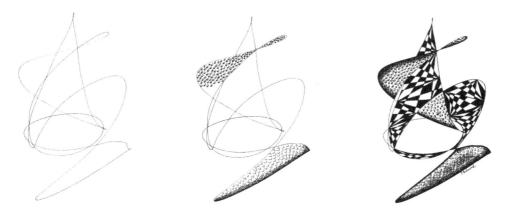

Be willing to let go of worry and allow your spirit to rest, recover and regroup one doodle at a time. Picasso said it best — "Art washes from the soul the dust of everyday life."

Everything you need to journey through those unexpected times in life is birthed out of the moment you're in NOW, not the moment down the road or the one you've already left behind.

[doodle and journal page]

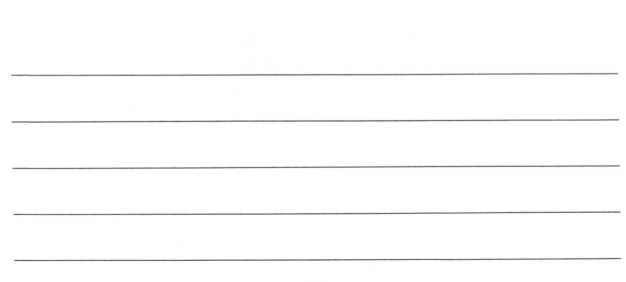

Doodling is an open-eyed meditation
where East meets West,
where fear meets faith,
and where the unknown
becomes known.

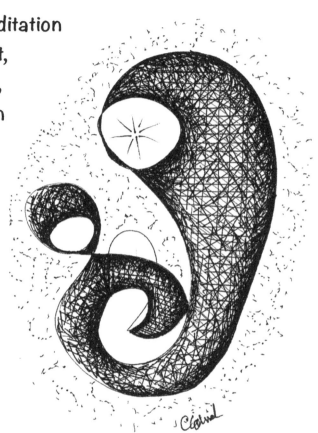

[doodle page]

If you can walk — you can dance.
If you can speak — you can sing.
If you can hold a pen in your hand —
you can doodle!

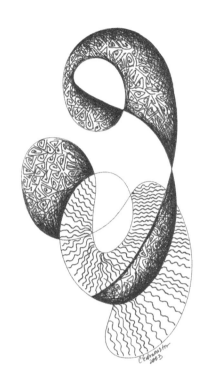

Have faith...
you truly receive no more
than you have the capacity to handle.

[doodle page]

Exploring the inner garden of life is about exploring that sacred space within, which ultimately dictates the quality of life we will experience in all that comes our way, especially when we find ourselves on an unexpected detour. Yet, even in the midst of the unexpected, we have within the capacity to rise to a new level — to elevate our state of being and align ourselves with the tools necessary to journey through challenging times.

It's more than just trying to seek the light at the end of the tunnel. It's about seeing the light along the way, and welcoming its presence into our hearts — into that inner garden as we're guided from beginnings, middles, and endings every day.

The goal is to become empowered in spite of the unexpected, as opposed to feeling victimized because of the unexpected. At times it may not feel like a cakewalk, but its well worth the effort in the long run.

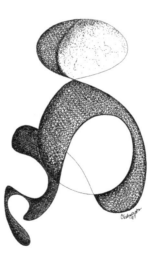

We are more than the sum of our thoughts, emotions and feelings, or worldly accomplishments. We are more than what we can see, touch, or feel. It's important to remember we are spiritual beings having a human experience, not the other way around, as French philosopher Pierre Teilhard de Chardin once said.

[doodle page]

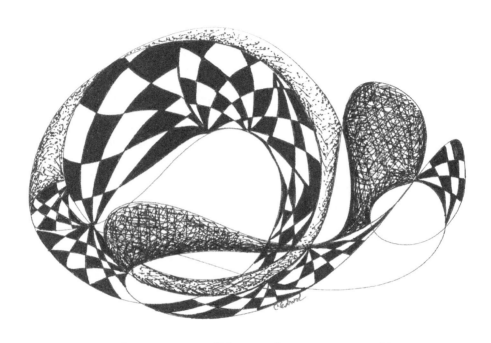

One must still have chaos in oneself
to be able to give birth to a dancing star...
—Nietzsche

[doodle page]

You have to accept whatever comes
and the only important thing is that you
meet it with the best you have to give...
–Eleanor Roosevelt

Life is about the sacred connections made
as you journey between two points.

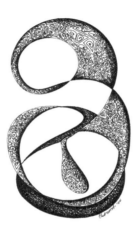

What are some of the sacred connections you've made along the way — those life adventures or events that brought about an "aha" moment? Some may have been unexpected and caught you by surprise, but you found a shining star, nonetheless.

_____

_____

_____

_____

_____

[doodle page]

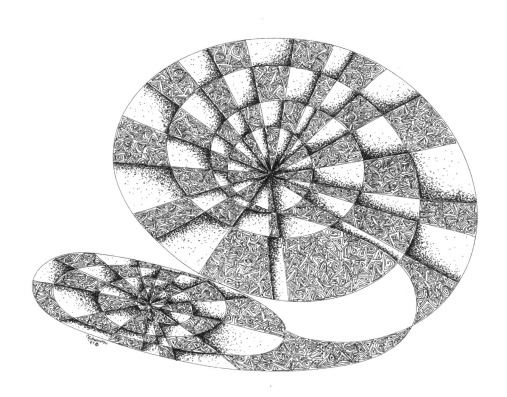

Life is a spiral journey of many different adventures,
with many different beginnings, middles and endings.
When one adventure ceases to exist, another begins.

[doodle and journal page]

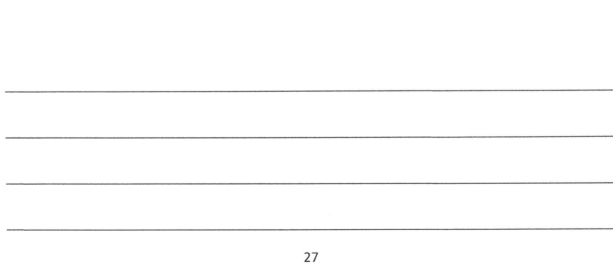

[doodle page]

In the middle of chaos hold on and remember,
it's all about faith. It's all about trust.

It's a myth to think the outer circumstances in life are the cause of our fears, stress, and anxiety. In truth, it's how we perceive things to be, and the choices made along the way.

Remember, the words you choose are very powerful. They are alive and filled with tremendous energy. Personally, I have never liked the term Breast Cancer SURVIVOR. I wanted to learn how to blaze a trail rather than just put out a fire. My mission was to learn how to thrive in spite of — to rise above a challenging chapter in my life and become transformed along the way.

I have invested over 11 million minutes in this spiritually rich, medical adventure. Learning how to thrive in spite of having my life temporarily turned upside down actually empowered me in ways I never imagined.

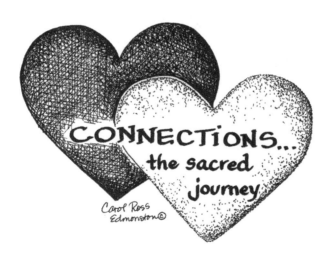

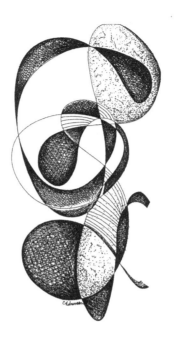

[doodle page]

[doodle page]

The world is a mere reflection
of one's inner vision of one's Self.
You see and experience life
as you see and experience yourself.

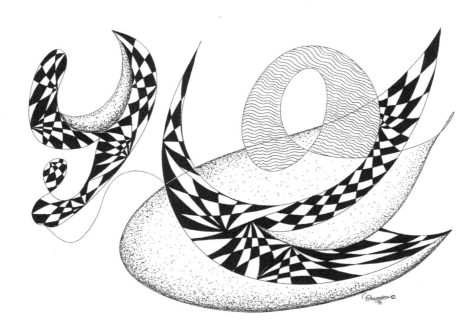

[doodle page]

A picture is not thought out and settled beforehand. While it is being done
it changes as one's thoughts change. And when it is finished, it still goes on
changing, according to the state of mind of whoever is looking at it...
–Picasso

Life is either a daring adventure
or nothing at all...
–Helen Keller

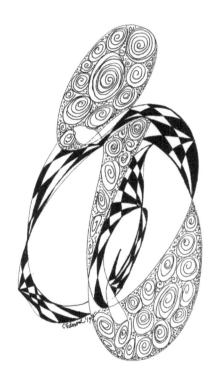

Beginnings, middles and endings are an interesting phenomena. After time a beginning becomes a middle, a middle becomes an ending, and an ending becomes a new beginning. They all come together to create a bigger story — the story of who we are through the ups and downs of everyday life. We're not one without the other. This is what makes for a great life — living and embracing all that comes our way.

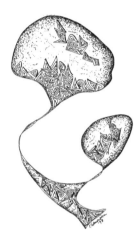

What's in your middle?

_____

_____

_____

_____

[doodle and journal page]

[doodle page]

If a man insisted always on being serious,
and never allowed himself a bit of fun
and relaxation, he would go mad...
—Herodotus

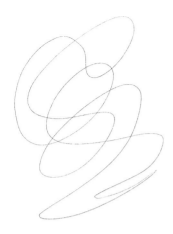 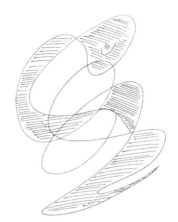 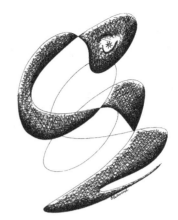

Just doodle... It's as easy as 1, 2, 3!

1. In one continuous motion, begin and end your doodle outline at the same point, without lifting the pen off the paper. Complete your outline in 5-7 seconds.

2. Fill in your doodle with anything that comes to mind — hearts, dots, circles, etc. Let your imagination guide you as you learn to trust the creative process.

3. Have fun and don't worry about what you create. Just have fun creating.

[doodle page]

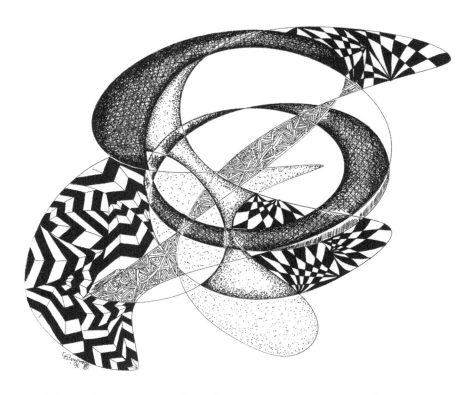

If you know exactly what you are going to do,
what's the good of doing it?
There's no interest in something you know already.
It's much better to do something else...
—Picasso

As you continue to doodle, are you finding it easier to relax and surrender to a spontaneous moment in time — to trust and have faith in the creative process with little regard to end result? If not, what did you experience? If your mind wandered to worldly concerns, take a deep breath in and long breath out and let your breath bring you back to a more calm and peaceful space.

_____

_____

_____

_____

[doodle page]

Now that you've completed a several doodles, take a few moments to notice if there is a parallel between your wandering mind while you doodle, and your wandering mind while you deal with challenging moments in your everyday life. Remember, an undisciplined mind can easily take you down a path filled with stress and anxiety.

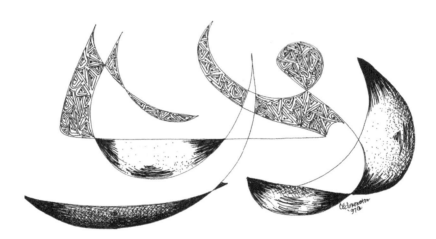

By anchoring yourself in a space of inner calm you can connect with your higher self and the wellspring of wisdom and innate sense of guidance to help you navigate through challenges of everyday life. This is the power of using doodling — a creative vehicle to bring you into an inner state of peace and stillness.

And...the good news is there are no mistakes when doodling!

Change your thoughts and you change your world...
–Norman Vincent Peal

Is it becoming easier for you to let go of the unknown tomorrows and stay focused in the present moment? If not, what obstacles are in the way?

_____

_____

_____

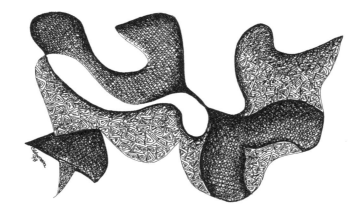

How to Journey Through Challenging Times...

1. Make a commitment to show up and become your own advocate.

2. Be willing to believe in yourself, even in the midst of outer chaos and confusion. Courage is the power to let go of the familiar and trust the unknown.

3. Nourish and nurture your spirit every day. Don't allow stress to dampen your spirit.

4. Remember, life begins at the end of your comfort zone. So when you find yourself on a detour, learn how to enjoy the scenery along the way.

5. Never give up! Life gives us no more than we have the capacity to handle. Trust the journey! Miracles happen when least expected.

[doodle page]

[doodle and journal page]

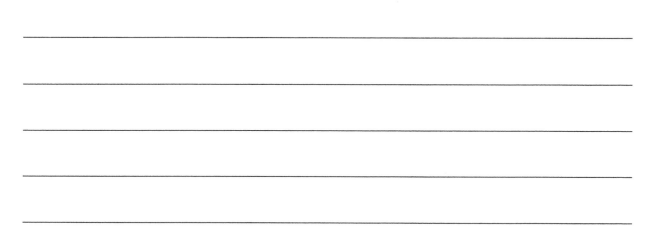

Now, take a moment and look through your finished doodles and notice all the different areas — at the top, bottom, sides and middle. Imagine each represents one of your life chapters or adventures. Perhaps some were filled with joy — the birth of a child, getting married or a job promotion. Perhaps some represented those more challenging times — those unexpected twists and turns that catch us off guard. However, when you put them all together and look at the big picture its hard to see anything less than a masterpiece — your unique masterpiece.

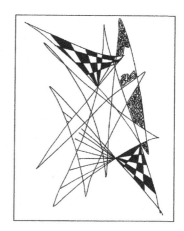

Each part came together to create the life you have now. When one ended, another began. They have built upon each other like a spiral. The important thing to remember is to not to allow any one event to dictate the quality of your life thereafter. For me, one of my greatest challenges was breast cancer. Yet, I was determined to turn that medical adventure into something greater — to discover the strength of who I am. In the end, the doodles I designed actually redesigned me from the inside out.

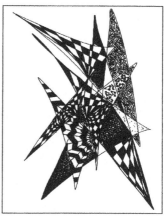

Doodling kept me so focused in the present moment — on the journey between two points — the initial diagnosis and end of treatment, and not on what "might" happen down the road.

Everything you need to journey through those unexpected times in life is birthed out of the moment you're in NOW, not the moment down the road or the one you've already left behind. Be willing to let go of worry and allow your spirit to rest, recover and regroup one doodle at a time.

Remember, the space between yesterday and tomorrow is where the divine world enters the human world. So take a deep breath in and a long breath out and Be Here Now!

The aim of art is to represent not the outward appearance
of things, but their inward significance...
—Aristotle

[doodle and journal page]

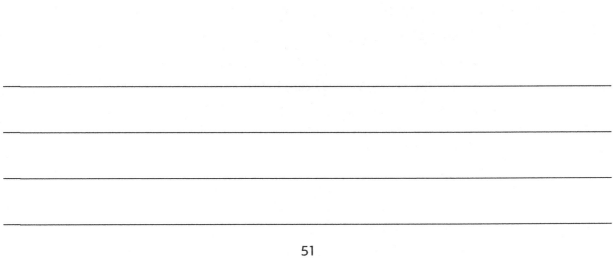

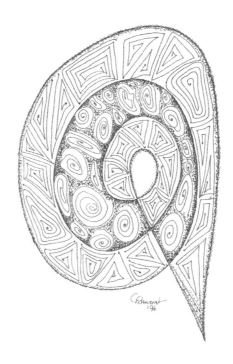

We live in a world of divinely inspired, orderly chaos.
We may not have a choice in what comes our way,
but we do have a choice in how we respond.
Learn how to turn obstacles into opportunities.
All moments are blessed — the good and the not as good.

[doodle and journal page]

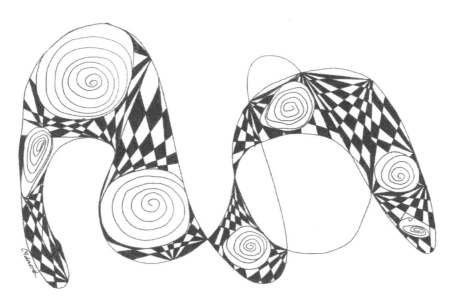

In the middle, life happens.
The past is gone and the future has yet to arrive.
Let go of the "if only's" from yesterday,
and the "what if's" from tomorrow
and be with "what is" in this moment in time.
Trust the journey!
The healing power of doodling is in the balancing
the lightness of creativity with the heaviness of life.

One today is worth two tomorrows...
-Benjamin Franklin

_____

_____

_____

_____

[doodle page]

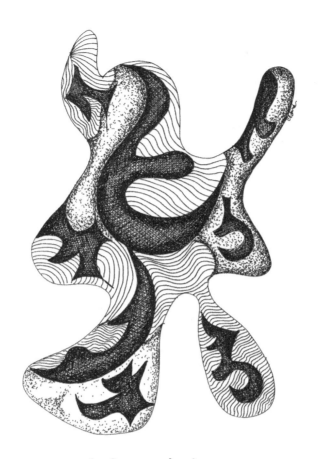

Life is a balance
of holding on
and letting go...
—Rumi

[doodle page]

We arrive at the place we started to be reminded
that we're here for the first time...
– T.S. Eliot

58

Every doodle is unique just like a snowflake — a one-of-a-kind. You don't need to compare it to anyone else's, or have it professionally analyzed. Simply take refuge in knowing your doodle reflected a peaceful present moment where you took the time to nourish and nurture your spirit.

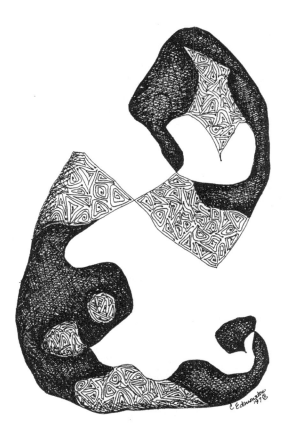

[doodle page]

Never let the present moment be merely a stepping stone to tomorrow.

What are some of the current life adventures going on in your world? Are you at peace with them, or do you find yourself struggling along the way? Do you have a positive strategy in place to help as you journey from day to day?

_____

_____

_____

_____

_____

_____

_____

_____

_____

[doodle page]

If you take away man's capacity to fear,
you also take away his capacity to grow...
-Rabbi Joshua L. Liebman

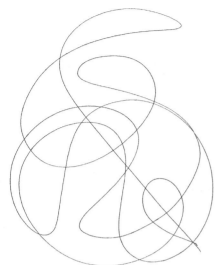

Remember...
life is about the sacred connections
made as you journey between two points.

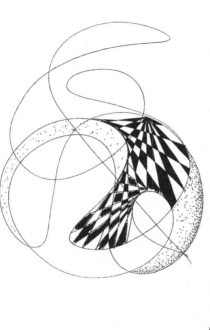

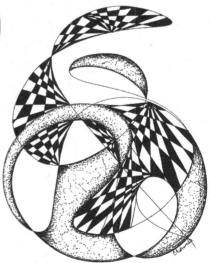

You're never too young to doodle!
Share the Sacred Doodles Method with your children.

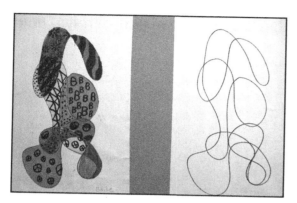 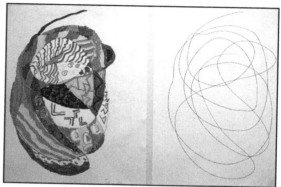

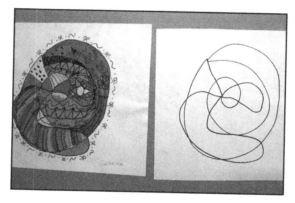

Doodle Art by 4th Grade Students

You're never too young to doodle!

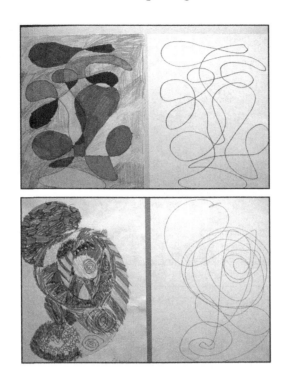

Doodle Art by 4th Grade Students

Every child is an artist.
The problem is how to remain an artist once he grows up...
–Picasso

Doodle Art by 4th Grade Student

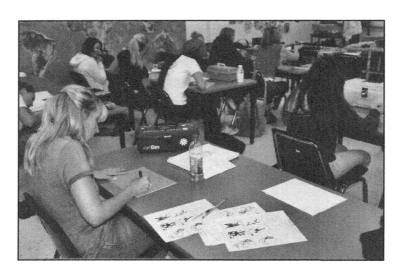

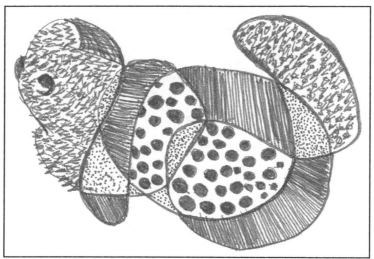

Doodle Art by 3rd Grade Students

Dear Mrs. Edmonston,

Thanks for teaching us about you uncle, Syd Hoff. I have read the book Danny and the Dionsaur and it was relt good. My most favorite part was when I saw the Doodle Art.

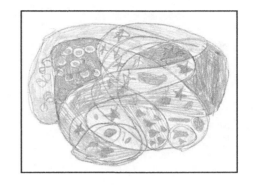

Dear Mrs. Edmonston,
Thank you for teaching us Doodle Art and your uncle Syd Hoff. My favorite part was when you showed us your Art in black and white beside. I LOVE your Art. f.y.i this is all in sei pen!

Love,
Dakoda #26

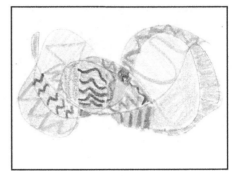

Dear Mrs. Edmonston,
Thank you for the lesine. I love all your art work it is asoume. Thankyou for teeching us about Syd hoff. I love when we did art. Love, Sonara Dec 18

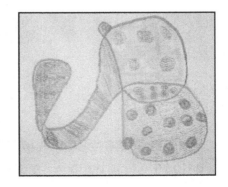

[kid's doodle page]
Be sure to sign your name and add a date

Remember — there are no mistakes when doodling.
Every doodle is unique — a one-of-a-kind, just like a snowflake!

[kid's doodle page]

Be sure to sign your name and add a date

Look to this day, for it is life.
For yesterday is but a dream and tomorrow is only a vision.
But today, well lived, makes yesterday a dream of happiness
and every tomorrow a vision of hope...
–Sanskrit Proverb

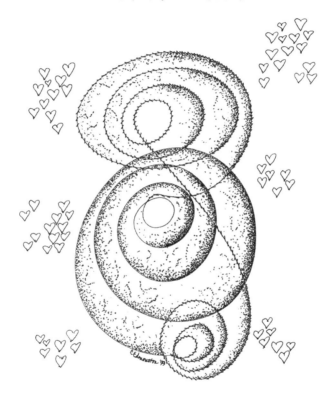

[doodle page]

Doodle Art Ideas:

1. Create your own doodle book, using a spiral-bound book filled with blank pages, and keep it with you as you journey throughout the day. This is a great family activity as well.

2. When you find yourself with some extra time, or feeling a bit stressed, take a few moments to "doodle" as a way to connect with a more calm inner space. You might also enjoy listening to soothing music, if possible. This can also help quiet and still your mind.

3. You can photocopy your doodles and make a lot of fun items, such as notecards and bookmarks. You can even frame your doodles with, or without, a mat, and give them as gifts or enjoy in your own home. Be sure to sign and date each doodle.

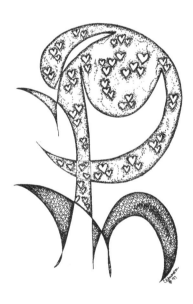

May the end of this book mark a new beginning for you
as you continue to experience the healing power of doodling
and the joy of living life one moment at a time.

Doodle Gallery

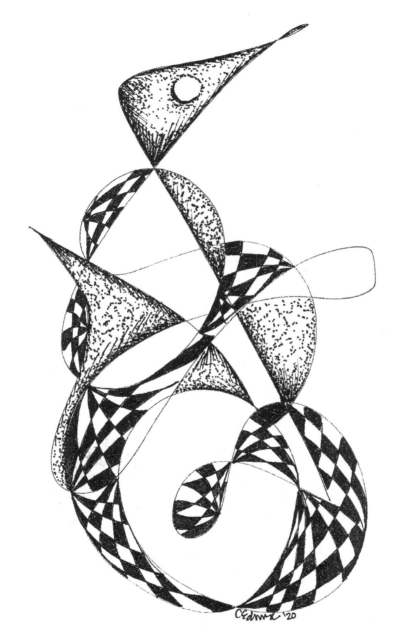

[doodle page]

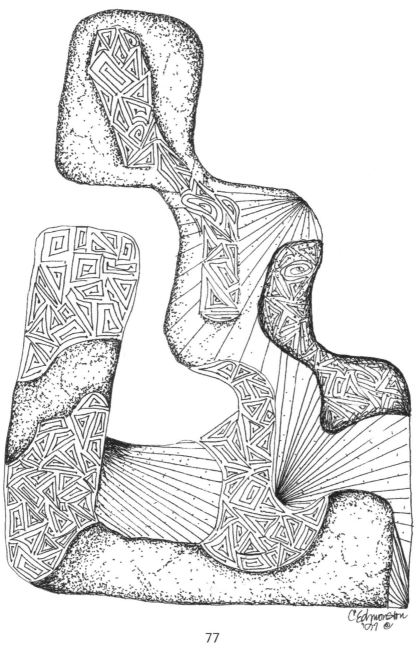

77

Creativity is intelligence having fun...
— Albert Einstein

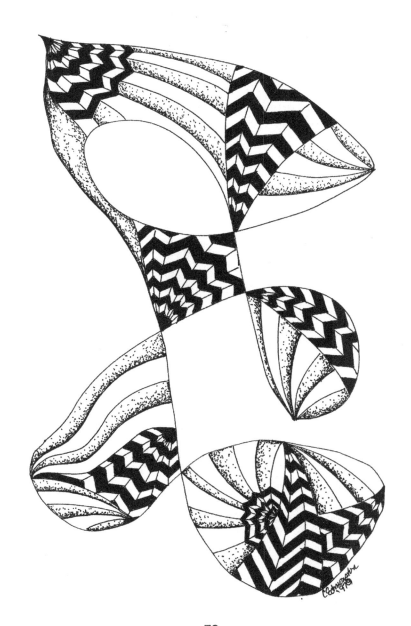

79

[doodle page]

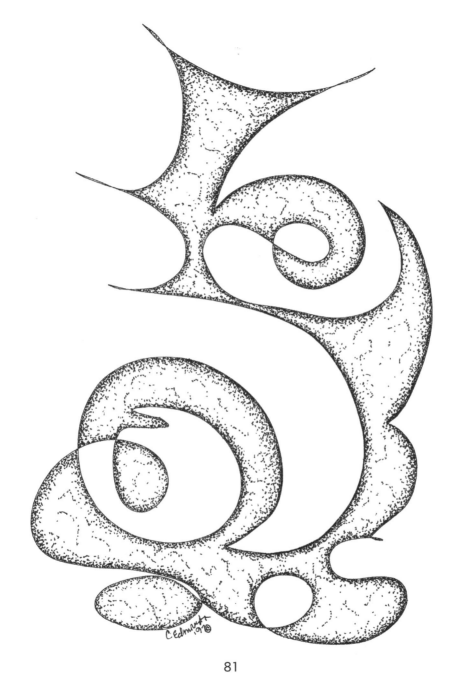

81

[doodle page]

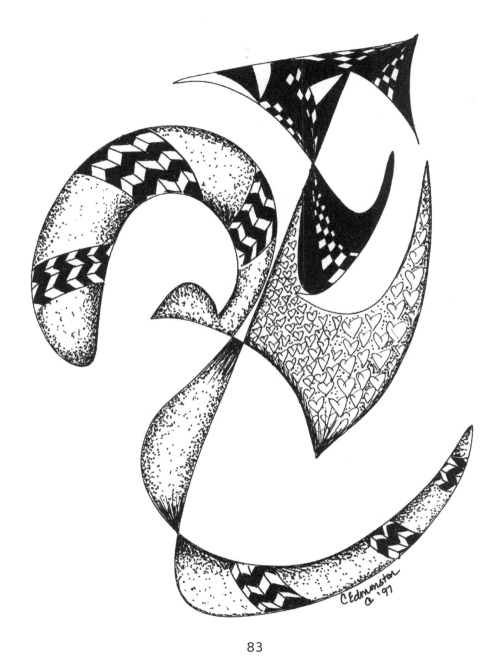

83

Sometimes your only means of transportation is a leap of faith...
— Margaret Vanderbilt Shepard

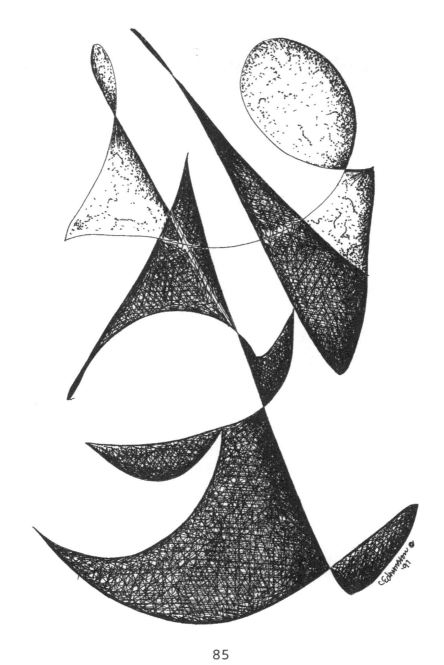

85

[doodle page]

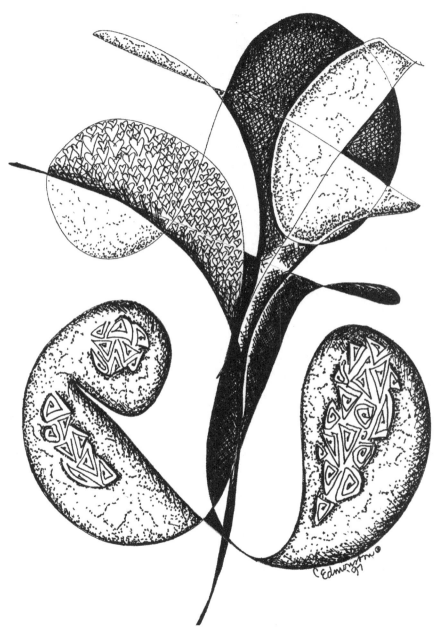

87

[doodle page]

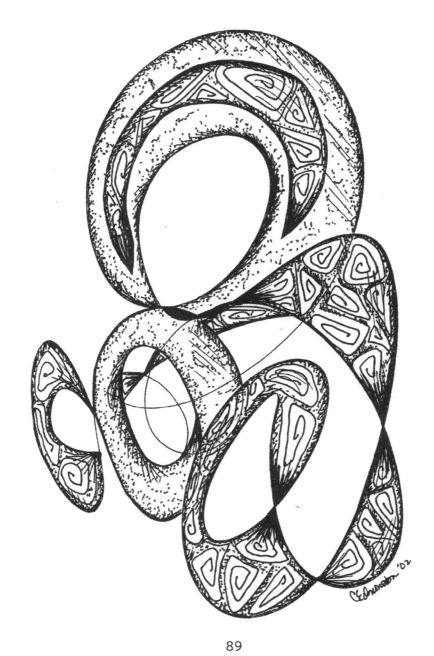

89

One of the secrets of life is to make stepping stones
out of stumbling blocks... —Jack Penn

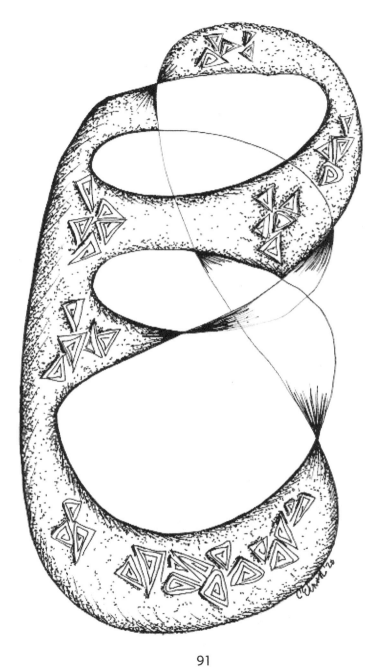

91

[doodle page]

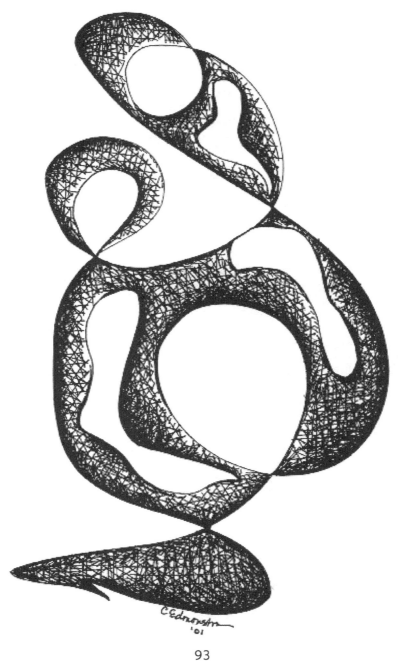

C.E.dmonson
'01

93

[doodle page]

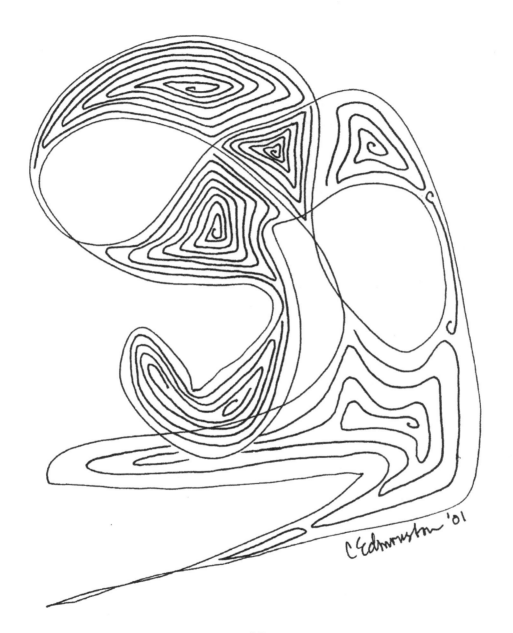

95

Our true home is to live in the present moment...
— Thich Nan Hahn

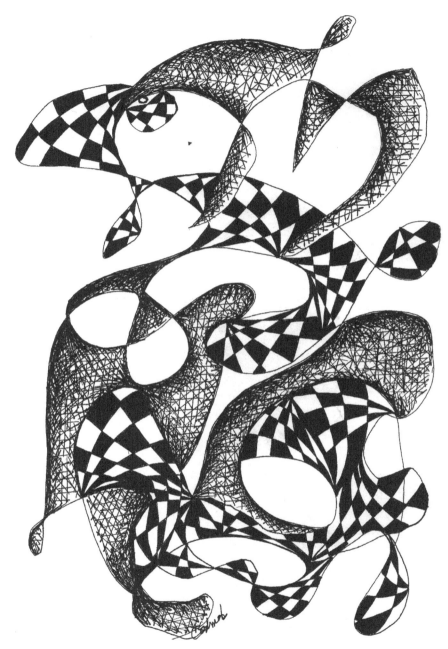

97

[doodle page]

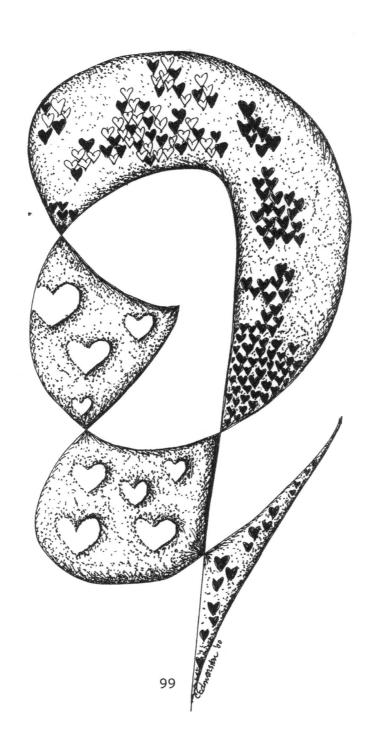

99

[doodle page]

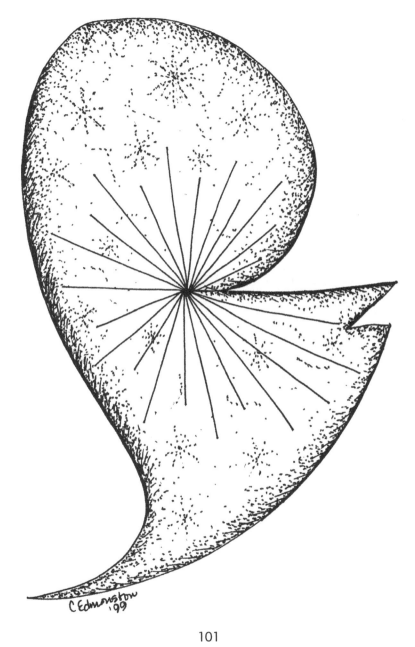

C Edmonston '99

You already have the precious mixture that will make you well—use it ...
— Rumi

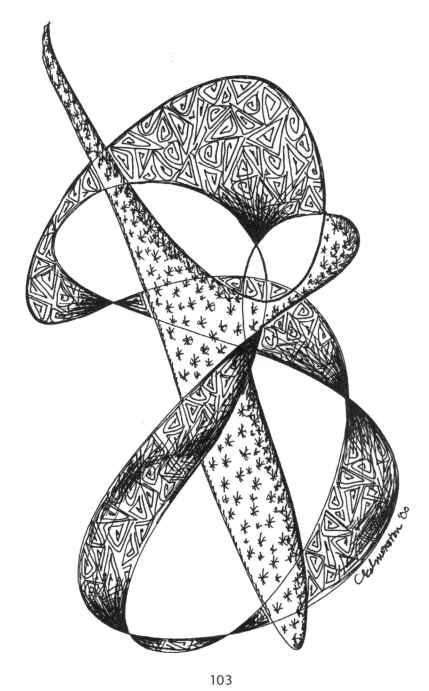

103

[doodle page]

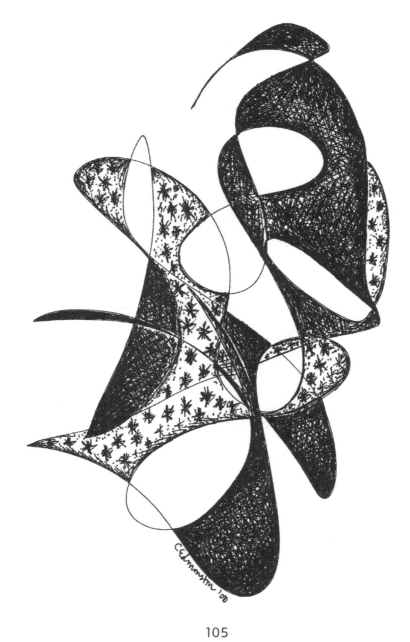

[doodle page]

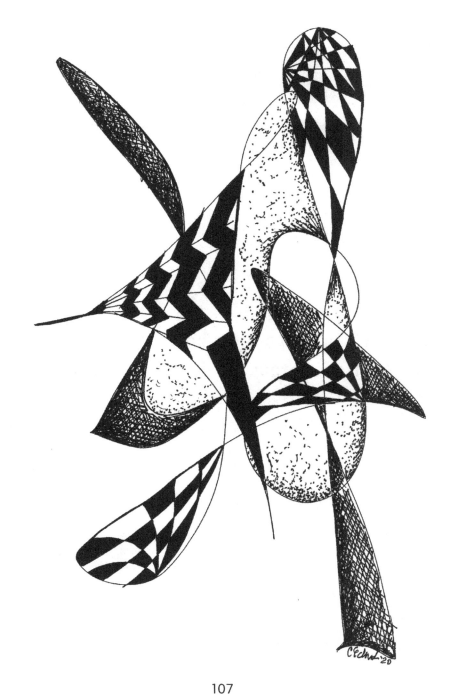

To practice any art, no matter how well or badly, is a way to make your soul grow. So do it... — Kurt Vonnegut

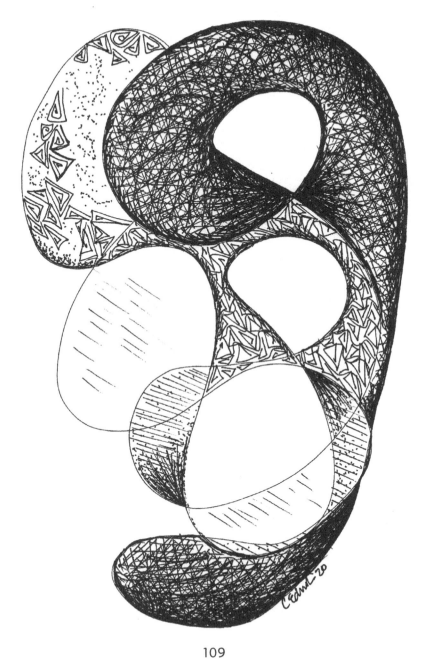

109

[doodle page]

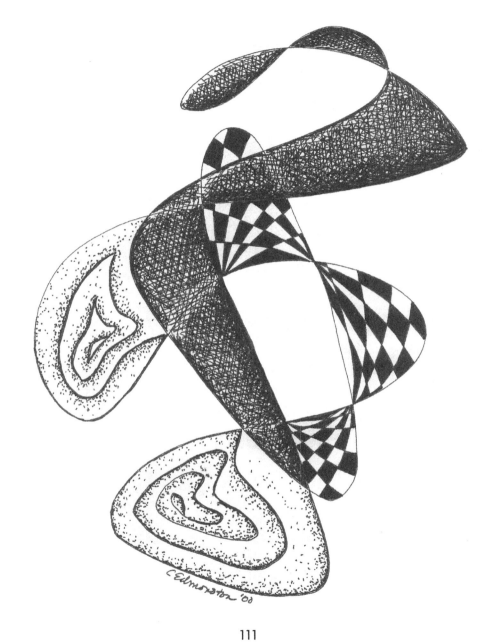

111

[doodle page]

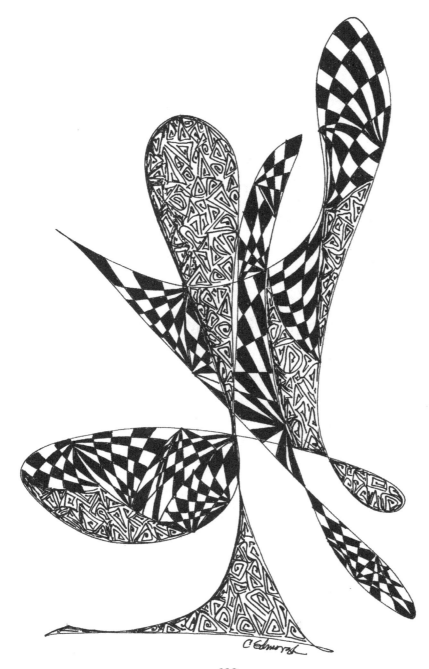

113

The best way out is through... — Robert Frost

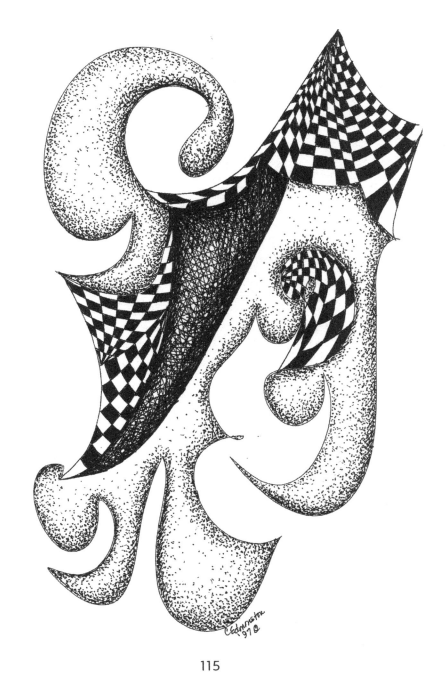

115

[doodle page]

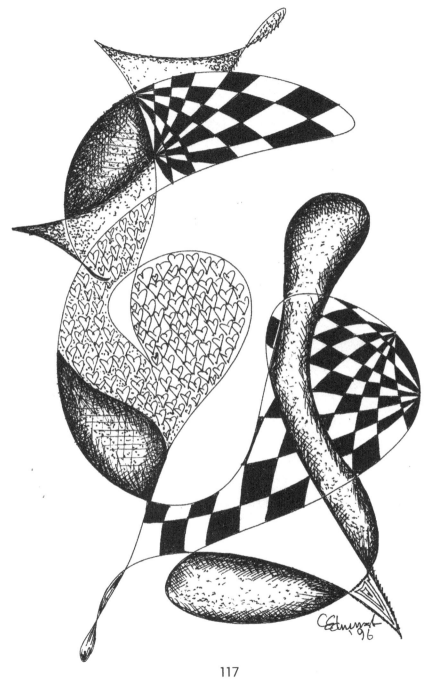

[doodle page]

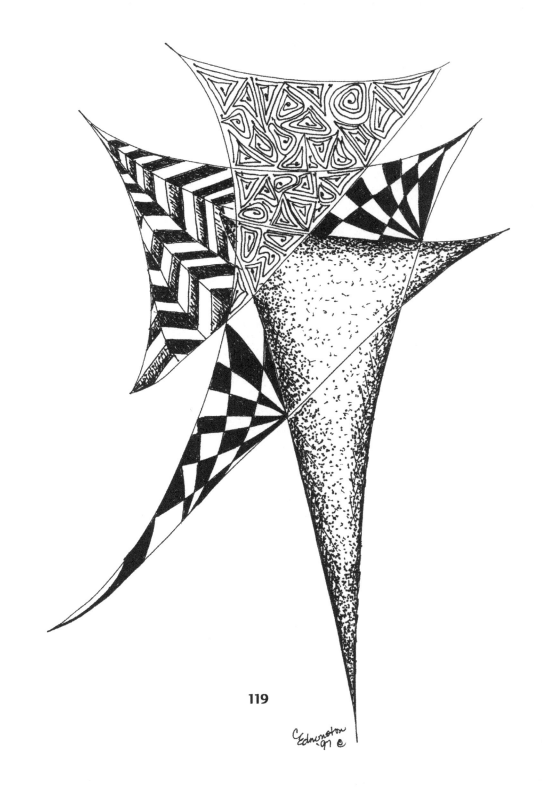

119

Edmonston '97 ©

Even the darkest night will end and the sun will rise...
— Victor Hugo

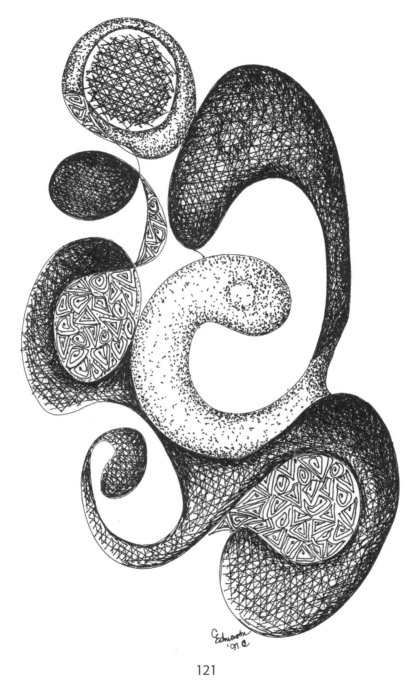

121

[doodle page]

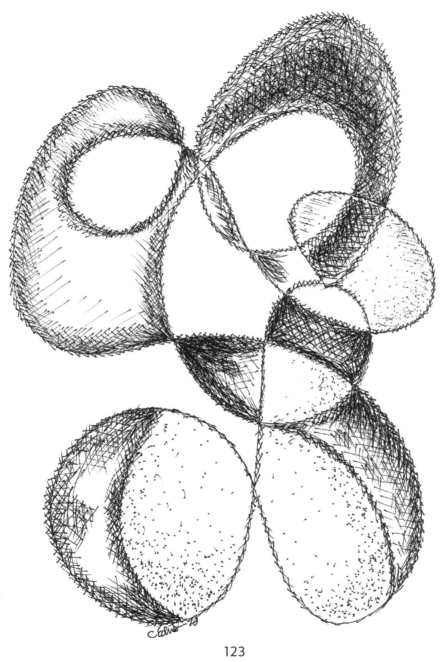

[doodle page]

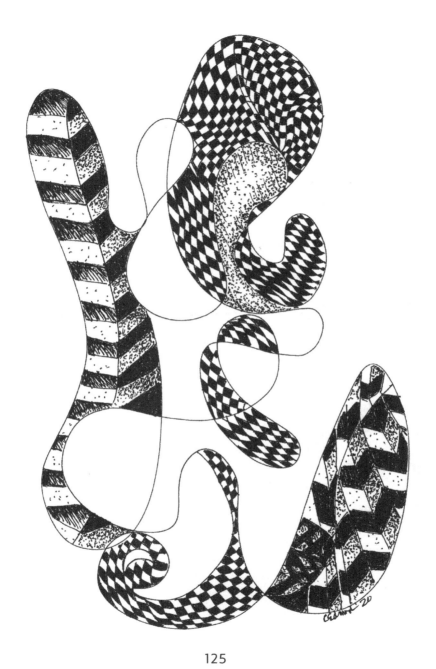

125

Start by doing what is necessary, then what is possible, and suddenly you are doing the impossible... — St. Francis of Assisi

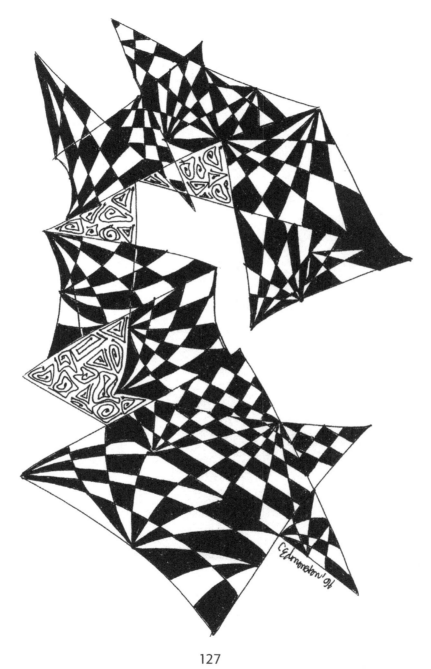

127

[doodle page]

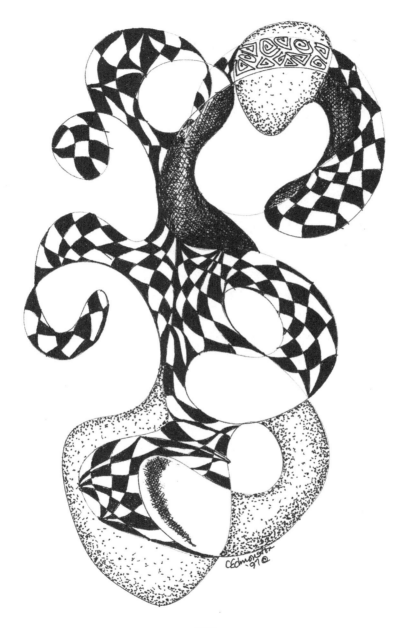

129

[doodle page]

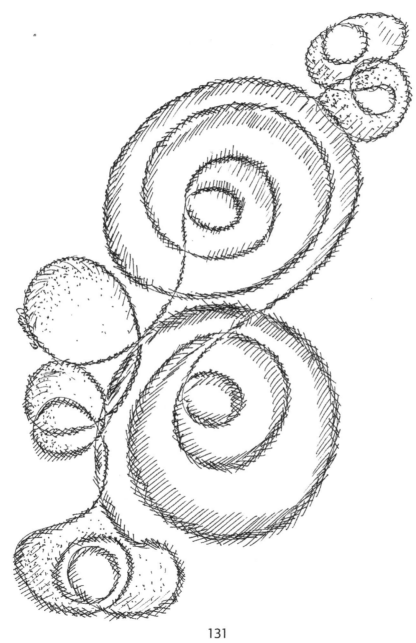

131

[doodle page]

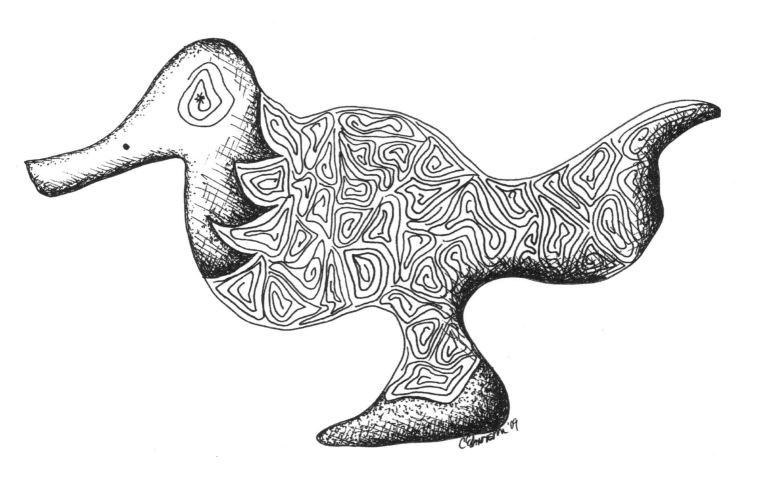

Be still, close your eyes, and turn your attention within. There is a perfect joy within the heart, a love like nectar—go there and find it. — Muktananda

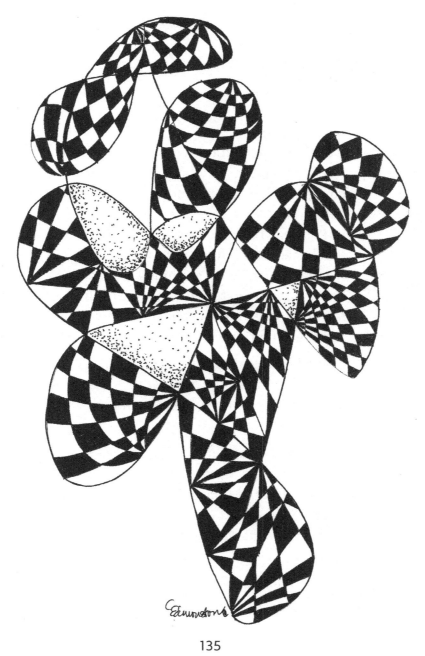

Edmonstone

135

About the Author

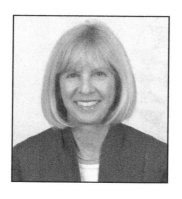

Carol Edmonston is an inspirational speaker known as The Doodle Lady™ who is committed to weaving together a connection between mind, body and spirit through the creativity of doodling. Born and raised in Los Angeles, Carol received her B.S. in Physical Therapy from the University of Southern California and became an author and speaker quite by accident. All it took was one suspicious mammogram and her world, the way she knew it, changed forever and she hasn't looked back since. Carol has conquered breast cancer, not once, but twice and shares her inspiring message with audiences of all ages from schools to health care settings.

Carol is the author three books: *The Healing Power of Doodling, Connections...the Sacred Journey between Two Points* and *Create While You Wait...a Doodle Book for All Ages.* Her DVD, entitled *Sacred Doodles,* weaves together her art and the Celtic harp sound of Lisa Lynne.

She has studied with some of the most influential thought leaders in the human potential movement, including Jean Houston and Caroline Myss, and a meditation master since 1988. Her story has been featured in *The Chicken Soup for Breast Cancers Survivor's Soul* and *The International Journal of Healing & Caring,* along with major media outlets, such as *The New York Times, Woman's World* and *Women's Health & Fitness.*

To learn more about workshops, speaking appearances, available art pieces and other helpful resources, visit SacredDoodles.com or TheDoodleLady.com. You can also find Carol on Facebook at The Original DoodleLady.

Made in the USA
Las Vegas, NV
08 April 2022